FITNESS SUTRA

WORKOUT FOR DESK BOUNDS

(REVISED 2ND EDITION)

Quick Stretches and Exercises to keep your Neck,
Shoulders, Back & Legs Pain-free and Mind
Active

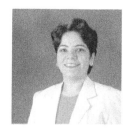

Dr. Monika Chopra
www.fitness-sutra.com

Dr. Monika Chopra's Fitness Sutra

Published by FitSutra Wellness Pvt Ltd,
33, Prachi Residency, Baner Rd., Pune-411045, India

ISBN-13: 978-1-6863-8792-0

Although I am a Physiotherapist (PT, for those of you in the USA) and a trained Yoga teacher, my suggestions through this book do not establish a doctor-patient relationship between us. This book is not intended to be a substitute for the medical advice of physicians. You should regularly consult a physician in matters relating to your health particularly with respect to any symptoms that may require diagnosis or medical attention. I advise you to take full responsibility of your safety and be aware of your physical limits. Before practising the exercises described in this book, be sure that your equipment is well maintained. Do not take risks beyond your level of flexibility, aptitude, strength, and comfort level.

This is a work of nonfiction. No names have been changed, no characters invented and no events fabricated. The information provided within this Book is for general informational purposes only. While I have tried to keep the information up-to-date and correct, there are no representations or warranties, expressed or implied, about the completeness, accuracy, reliability, suitability or availability with respect to the information, products, services, or related graphics contained in this book for any purpose. Any use of this information is at the reader's own responsibility. I do not assume and hereby disclaim any liability to any party for any loss, damage, or disruption caused by errors or omissions, whether such errors or omissions result from negligence, accident, or any other cause.

Foreword

I come across numerous patients with diseases that are outcome of a modern, desk bound and stressful lifestyle. Most of these could have been prevented simply by living a physically active life.

This book is a solution towards making your sedentary life active without altering your daily routines too much. With her sound knowledge of Physiotherapy and Yoga, Dr. Monika Chopra has done justice to her subject.

The exercises mentioned herein are simple and holistic. The routines are effective and would certainly help in improving your overall health and wellbeing.

Dr. K. H. Sancheti
Founder President and Chief Orthopedic Surgeon
Sancheti Institute for Orthopedics & Rehabilitation, Pune

Foreword by Author

I would like to thank you and congratulate you for buying this book. This book will definitely guide you to a "*healthy you*" in light of the exercises suggested.

In more than a decade of working as a physical therapist and a holistic lifestyle consultant, I have come across lot of people suffering from the occupational hazards of long work hours and a sedentary lifestyle. The list of problems start from back ache, shoulder pains, carpal tunnel syndrome, and cervical pain; stretching over to knee pain, varicose veins, and ankle & heel pains. Most of these problems are associated with problems of low concentration spans, anxiety, stress, depression and obesity. A connection between all these problems is obvious and is the outcome of ignoring our physical and mental health. This is due to long working hours, short break times, lack of exclusive workouts and the immense pressures of meeting work commitments coupled with faulty eating habits.

Unfortunately work cultures and practices are often not very heart friendly, weight observant or mentally healthy. Similar to a home, social gatherings or school, the workplace has some norms and unwritten rules that everyone is expected to follow. Nobody wants to be known as a coffee guzzling whale or a cigarette junkie at the workplace. Nor is it considered professional if a person gets up every 45 minutes or an hour to go for a walk outside. Though all norms and regulations are made to improve productivity and efficiency at the workplace, they don't really work in favor of our health and hence affect our work output indirectly (& directly if left ignored).

It's about time we make subtle changes in our working style and routine so that we can have a healthy mind and a healthy body which in turn will improve our productivity and efficiency at the workplace.

Acknowledgments

This book would not have been possible without the confidence of my clinical patients. They have put faith in me, followed my instructions to the letter and provided me great feedback about the efficacy and usefulness of each exercise mentioned in these pages.

I especially thank my dear friends Vijayshree Abhyankar & Yuvraj Pingale for taking time out of their busy schedules and creating the perfect illustrative pictures for the first edition of this book – "Exercises with Deep Breathing for Sedentary Lifestyles". The illustrations presented in the current edition draw heavily upon their contribution.

Last, but not the least, I thank my family, whose unquestioning support continues to be pillar of my strength.

CONTENTS

1   What to Expect From This Book?   1

2   The Sitting Epidemic   4

3   Correct Posture for a Healthy Body   9

4   Exercises for Cervical Region   17
    Neck Rotations   18
    Neck Isometrics   20
    Seated Neck Stretches   23

5   Exercises for Shoulder Region   26
    Shoulder Rotations   27
    Forward Arm Stretch   30
    Upward Arm Stretch   32
    Backward Arm Stretch   34

6   Exercises for Arms, Shoulders & Upper Back   36
    T Arms Rotation   36
    Triceps Dips   38
    Biceps Curls   40
    Self-Handshake   42
    W Arms Retraction   44

7   Exercises for the Wrists & Hands   46
    Wrist Extensions   47
    Wrist Rotations   49

8   Exercises for Chest   51
    Namaste   52
    Wall Push-Ups   53

Desk Cat & Camel Stretches   55

9   Exercises for Back Relaxation   57
    Forward Bends in Sitting Position   58
    Figure of Four Forward Bend   60
    L Shaped Body Stretch   62
    Seated Spine Twists   64
    Standing Side Bends   66
    Standing Backwards Bend   68

10   Exercises for the Abdomen   70
    Secret Tummy Tucks   71
    Chair Crunches   72
    Chair Swivels   74
    Chair Forward and Backward Movements   76

11   Exercises for Lower Body   78
    Seat Squeezes   79
    Leg Raises   80
    Desk Squats   82
    Standing Leg Curls   84
    Inner Thigh Squeezes   86
    Tap into Toes   88
    Jog in Your Place   89
    Calf Raises   90
    Standing Leg Raises – Sideward   92
    Standing Leg Raises - Forwards &   94
Backwards

12   Shake the Tension Off   96
    Fist Punches   96
    Flapping Arms   98
    Axe Movement   99

13 Progressive Muscle Relaxation   101

14 Breath Awareness   105

15 Supported Surya Namaskar   111

16 Final Tips   120

17 Eye Exercises   122

18 Bonus   124

CHAPTER 1

What to Expect From This Book?

This book is a practical guide on how to balance your busy work schedules with a sound exercise regime.

Exercises should not be kept as a monthly or yearly agenda but should be made an integral part of your lifestyle. To be physically and mentally healthy you don't always need huge green lawns to walk on or to spend a fortune on expensive gym memberships and personal trainers. Neither is it necessary to consume tons of flashy supplements and nutrition pills.

By following a thoughtful lifestyle and consciously and religiously doing the simple exercises mentioned in this book, you can achieve a healthy mind in a healthy body, right in the confines of your workplace.

You may already be well informed on the following tips of healthy living,

1. Consuming lots of vegetables and fruits as they are rich in vitamins and minerals and low in calories as compared to animal based foods.

2. Minimizing the consumption of empty calories present in fast food.

3. Minimizing the consumption of preserved and packaged food which is high on sugar & sodium content and low on potassium, that the body needs to maintain electrolyte balance.

4. Drinking a minimum of 8-10 glasses of water daily. Two thirds of our body is made of water. Water acts as a carrier for nutrients, regulates body temperature and detoxifies the body.

5. Staying away from smoking and alcohol consumption.

6. Getting enough sleep of 7-8 hours every night to optimize mental and physical energy and improve longevity.

7. Getting plenty of sunlight which helps in synthesizing Vitamin D in our body which in turn has a wide spectrum of benefits such as improved immunity and decreased risks of cancer, heart disease, multiple sclerosis and osteoporosis.

This book aims to make you realize that

1. Your body is the most important workout tool you have.

2.   You don't need tons of complicated equipment and methods to feel energetic and fit.

3.   Your workplace can act as your workout area without compromising on your work ethics or needing to reschedule your busy meeting hours.

4.   Practice of breathing techniques and meditation can help decrease anxiety and stress and improve concentration.

5.   Your weight loss starts in your mind. With steely willpower you can lose up to 15 pounds in less than two months of sitting in your cubicle.

And most importantly, you can enjoy the fruits of your hard work in the long term by avoiding getting struck by chronic lifestyle diseases like obesity, heart attacks, diabetes, hypertension etc., by engaging in these simple exercises.

CHAPTER 2

The Sitting Epidemic

Mostly sedentary lifestyle of today is one of the biggest culprits of health deterioration. While some experts are calling the sedentary lifestyle and its ill-effects as "*The Sitting Disease*"; I term it as an *Epidemic*. A vast majority of patients at my Physical Therapy practice find sedentary lifestyle as the biggest root cause of their ailments, even after discounting for the ill-effects of drinking, smoking, eating fast food etc. If we observe our daily routine, we will realize how most of our day is spent on our hind and not on the feet (as our bodies have evolved in nature). Be it watching TV, eating food, commuting, working in the cubicle, chatting with friends, watching a game; we are sitting all the time. The only breaks from sitting are when we are forced to walk short distances, typically between one siting spot to another like moving from the parking to office.

Thus we spend a major part of our day in a sedentary manner. Sitting affects our body negatively in the following ways

Damaging Body Organs

1. <u>Heart Disease</u>: Sitting for long hours decreases fat burn by muscles and blood flow in the body, predisposing the heart to fatty acid clog. Prolonged sitting elevates blood cholesterol levels and leads to high blood pressure. No wonder people with

sedentary lifestyle are twice more prone to cardio vascular diseases.

2. <u>Over-productive Pancreas</u>: Pancreas produces insulin, a hormone that carries glucose to cells for energy. Sitting for longer durations makes a lot of muscles idle and the cells in idle muscles don't respond well to insulin (this is also called insulin resistance). As a result the pancreas produces more and more insulin, leading to diabetes and other diseases.

3. <u>Non-alcoholic Fatty Liver Disease</u>: Increasing insulin resistance is also linked to development of Non-alcoholic Fatty Liver Disease which can lead to liver cirrhosis, also known as chronic liver damage. This causes healthy liver tissues to be replaced by scar tissues. Liver is the second largest and one of the most complex organs in the body. It is a key organ of the digestive system. The liver plays a crucial role in fighting infections and diseases, regulating blood sugar levels, removing toxins from the body, in addition to controlling cholesterol levels and helping blood to clot. A damaged liver is unable to discharge these vital life functions effectively.

4. <u>Colon, Breast & Endometrial Cancer</u>: Prolonged sitting can lead to colon, breast and endometrial cancer. Though the reason is unclear, there are two theories around this. Firstly, increased insulin encourages abnormal cell growth and thus causes cancer. Secondly, lesser range of movement

decreases natural anti-oxidants in the body. These anti-oxidants are responsible for killing cell damaging and cancer causing free radicals. With their suppression, free radicals reign free in the body, increasing the chances of cancer.

5. Pulmonary Embolism in Lungs: Sedentary lifestyle causes formation of blood clots which can travel to lungs leading to pulmonary embolism (characterized by shortness of breath and chest pain).

6. Muddled Brain: Active muscles improve oxygenated blood flow to the brain. This triggers the release of brain and mood enhancing chemicals, thus making you mentally and physically active. Inactive muscles cannot activate the release of these natural mood elevating chemicals leading to either a muddled brain or a gradually developing dependence on chemicals (like nicotine and other psychedelic substances).

Muscle Degeneration

1. Weak Abs: Abdominal muscles (i.e. abs) play an important role in maintaining an erect standing or sitting posture. A long hour of sitting in a slumped position puts your abs to disuse, ultimately leading to a weak core. A weak core further gives way to an exaggerated lumbar spine arch (hyperlordosis) causing back aches.

2. <u>Tight Hip Flexors</u>: Hips form a very important part of the locomotor system. Hip flexibility is essential for standing, walking, maintaining balance and a proper posture. Sitting for longer durations leads to hip flexor (i.e. muscles in front of hips) tightness and limit the range of motion and stride. Tight hip flexors increase anterior pelvic tilt, thus exaggerating the lumbar curve.

3. <u>Limp Glutes</u>: Glutes (i.e. hip extensor muscles or Gluteus muscles) aren't in use while sitting, which makes them weak. Glutes help in standing up from a sitting position, and propelling the body to a stride. Hence weak glutes affect body balance and strength adversely.

Problems Affecting Legs

1. <u>Poor Blood Circulation in Legs</u>: Sitting for long hours decreases the blood circulation in legs leading to fluid pooling. This can cause varicose veins, swollen legs and deep vein thrombosis.

2. <u>Weak/Soft Bones</u>: Weight bearing activities like walking and running stimulate the lower limb bone growth, making them stronger, thicker and denser. Prolonged sitting deprives the body of this activity and causes weaker bones and osteoporosis.

Trouble in Upper Body

1. Strained Neck: Long hours of working in front of computers can strain the cervical region leading to cervical spondylosis, neck pain and neck stiffness.

2. Sore Shoulder & Upper Back Pain: Neck pain is also accompanied with shoulder and upper back pain, slouching of upper back and shoulder and tingling sensations in arms and shoulders.

Back Problems

1. Stiff Spine: Long sitting hours cause stiffening of the spine. The inter-vertebral gap decreases, squashing the discs unevenly. With exercises, the para-spinal muscles strengthen, maintaining the inter-vertebral gap. The discs in the spine contract and expand with movement thus absorbing fresh blood and nutrients.

2. Prolapsed Disc / Herniated Lumbar Disc: Increased lumbar curve puts uneven pressure on the discs causing prolapsed discs.

Taking standing and exercise breaks after every 30/60 minutes can reduce the risk of above mentioned problems. You should do the simple stretches/exercises suggested in subsequent chapters over the course of the day and keep yourself active and healthy.

CHAPTER 3

Correct Posture for a Healthy Body

Posture is described as the carriage of the body as a whole, the attitude of the body, or the position of the limbs (the arms and legs).

What is a Good Posture?

There is no one, fixed body stance to describe good posture. A good posture is one in which the person's body is optimally aligned in such a way that the muscles can perform actions, requiring the least amount of energy to achieve the desired effect. While standing, good posture is when the body is natural, comfortable, aligned and balanced and not rigid and straight. While sitting, good posture is when the head, shoulder and trunk are aligned and back is comfortably straight. Good standing and sitting postures help promote normal functioning of the body's organs and increase the efficiency of the muscles, thereby minimizing fatigue.

Importance of Good Posture

1. Health: Good posture is essential to keep neck and back pain free. When we habitually sit, stand or walk in a less than fully aligned position, muscles stretch or contract to accommodate the imbalance, leading to back and neck pain. Holding the head, shoulders and trunk in perfect alignment increases

the efficiency of the muscles, thereby minimizing fatigue.

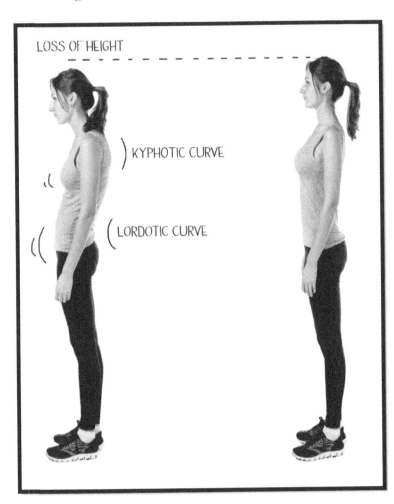

Good posture allows our many physiological systems to function optimally. Poor posture can often contribute to digestive, respiratory and cardiopulmonary problems over time.

2. Performance: Strong posture and balance is must for optimal athletic performance, whether it is for competitive, recreational or daily life activity purpose. Training core stabilization, fluid coordinated motion, balance and good posture are essential to promote movement efficiency and endurance and avoid injury.

3. Appearance: Your posture is what the world sees in you first. Posture affects mood, energy and self-confidence, all of which affect how attractive we appear to others. Your posture is your signature in *body language*. People with strong posture look better, more appealing, younger, more radiant, trimmer, and are perceived to be more confident.

Through vigilant maintenance of a correct posture, extra strain on the body can be reduced, thus bringing the related problems under control and also preventing their reoccurrence. Relaxation, mobility and strengthening exercises work wonders in maintaining a healthy static and dynamic posture.

Correct Standing Posture:

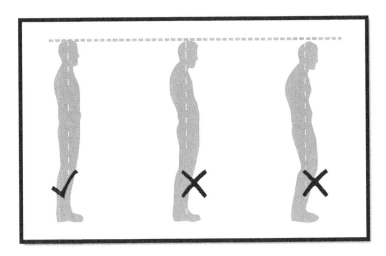

It is important to maintain the natural curve of the spine when standing. One should follow these guidelines while standing straight

1. Stand with the feet hip-width distance apart.
2. Outer edges of the feet should be parallel to each other.
3. Keep your knees slightly flexed, thigh muscles and buttocks contracted.
4. The spine should be erect with shoulders relaxed.
5. The chin should be parallel to the floor with neck straight for correct neck alignment.

For relaxed standing, follow the guidelines 3, 4, 5 with feet slightly apart, one foot in front of the other and knees slightly flexed. Use a box or slightly elevated area to prop one foot up while standing. Change feet position every 20 minutes.

Correct Sitting Posture:

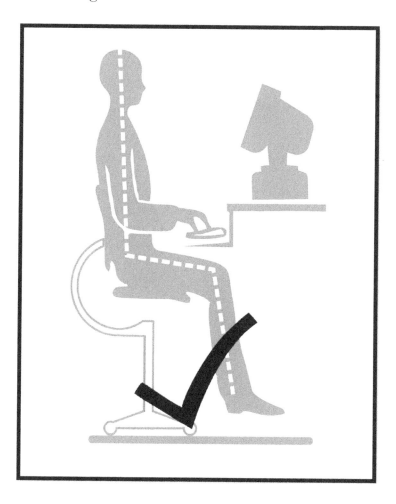

Many problems which arise because of long sitting hours can be avoided by adopting a proper sitting posture. Follow the below tips for a good sitting posture.

1. Keep your neck straight, while siting.
2. The top of your screen (if you are using a computer) should be at 10 degrees to your eye level.
3. Shoulders should be relaxed while working (avoid hunchback and shrugging of the shoulders).
4. Your forearms should be parallel to the floor while working.
5. The chair should have a backrest to support your back.
6. The seat should completely support your thigh.
7. There should be some gap between the edge of your seat and the back of your knee.
8. Your legs should be bent 90-110 degrees while sitting.
9. Sit straight with feet flat on the floor or supported by a footrest.
10. Take a break for stretching every 30 minutes.

Correct Driving Posture:

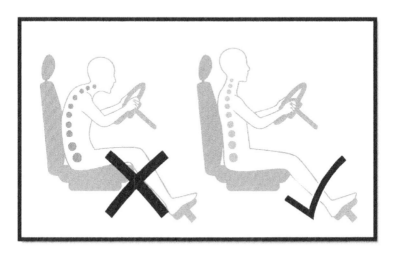

1. Always sit with your knees levelled with the hips.
2. A rolled up towel or a back support cushion can be placed behind the back for proper support.
3. Sit as close to the steering wheel as possible because reaching for it increases the pressure on the lumbar and cervical spine, shoulder and wrist.

Bonus

I hope you are finding this book useful and are ready to start with the exercises.

I have also created easy to use quick reference chart of these exercises, which can be placed at your desk for quick reference. This would also serve as a handy reminder to do your stretches at regular interval.

You can download the printable file from

https://www.fitness-sutra.com/go?id=111020

 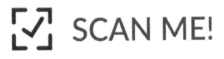

You can also subscribe to my mailing list to get more tips & motivation to do these exercises.

CHAPTER 4

Exercises for Cervical Region

The cervical region (neck) begins at the base of the skull and connects to the thoracic spine (upper back) through a series of seven cervical vertebral segments.

The neck is a delicate and well-engineered structure of bones, muscles, nerves, ligaments and tendons. It houses the spinal cord that sends messages from the brain to control all functions of the body. Along with this, it is a strong and flexible organ - allowing multidirectional movement. It supports the head, which on an average weighs 5 to 8 Kilograms. The vertebral openings in the cervical spine provide a passageway for vertebral arteries ensuring proper blood flow to the brain.

Cervical pain (cervical spondylosis) is one of the most common problems faced by people working long hours. It may start as mild, deep or severe pain in neck region, spreading to the shoulders and arms. It might be associated with stiffness in the neck, tingling sensations or numbness in the shoulders and arms, radiating to the fingers. This is usually accompanied by headaches.

The exercises mentioned in this chapter help to strengthen the neck muscles & also break the build-up of stress, through stretching.

Neck Rotations

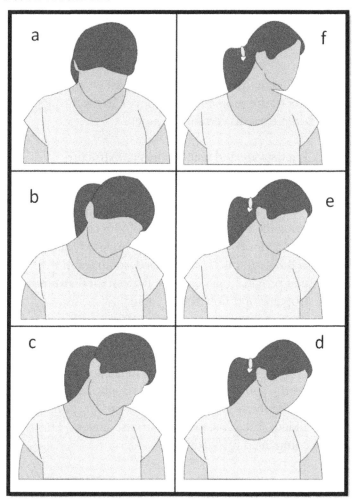

Effect: Releases tension in the neck. Stretches neck muscles and relieves muscle spasms. Improves neck mobility and flexibility. Alleviates headaches.

Important: Practice carefully in case of neck injuries.

Start Position: Sitting or standing straight with the spine erect, shoulders relaxed, chin parallel to the floor and looking straight ahead.

Steps:
1. Take your chin down towards the front of your chest. Exhale while doing this to feel a pleasant stretch behind your neck.
2. Rotate the neck & take your chin towards the left shoulder as you inhale. Look over your left shoulder. You should feel the stretch in the right side of your neck.
3. Rotate the neck bringing your chin back to the chest position as you exhale to feel the stretch behind your neck again.
4. Rotate the neck taking chin to the right shoulder as you inhale. Look over your right shoulder to feel the stretch on the left side of your neck.
5. Rotate the neck and bring the chin back to the chest position as you exhale. You should feel the stretch behind the neck.
6. Raise your chin as you inhale to get in the starting position.
7. Repeat the above sequence three times.

Fine Tips:
1. The neck rotation should be slow and rhythmic.
2. Keep your spine straight and chest outwards and lifted as you do these movements.
3. Movements must be done with breath awareness, feeling the muscles stretch and relax.

Neck Isometrics

In most individuals aged around 30-45 years, the predisposing cause of cervical spondylosis is the decrease in the distance between the cervical vertebrae joints which may occur because of misaligned posture during long working hours. Neck isometrics help to strengthen the neck muscles, thus helping one to maintain proper neck posture and prevent the onset of cervical spondylosis.

Effect: Strengthens the postural neck muscles giving better support to the neck. Releases tension in the neck. Helps to decrease symptoms of cervical spondylosis like chronic neck pain, radicular pain, diminished range of motion, headaches, weakness and impaired fine motor coordination.

Important: Practice carefully in case of neck Injuries.

Start Position: Sitting or standing straight with the spine erect, shoulders relaxed, chin parallel to the floor. Look straight ahead while preforming this exercise.

Steps:

Isometric Flexion
1. Place both hands with fingers interlocked on your forehead. Gently push both the hands and the forehead against each other, resisting the movement.
2. Hold for five counts and release.
3. Keep breathing as you perform the exercise.
4. Repeat five times.

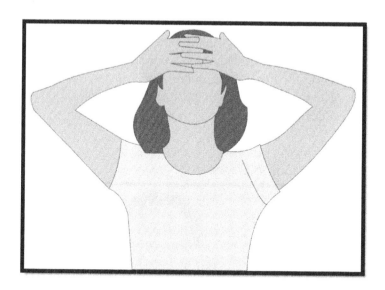

Isometric Extension

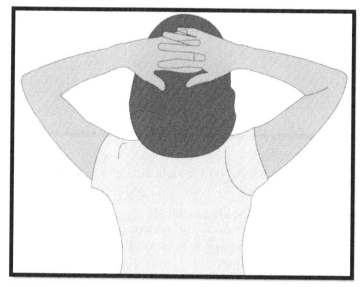

1. Place both hands with fingers interlocked behind the head. Push your hands and the skull against each other, resisting the movement.
2. Hold for five counts and release.
3. Keep breathing as you perform the exercise.
4. Repeat five times.

Isometric right Lateral Flexion

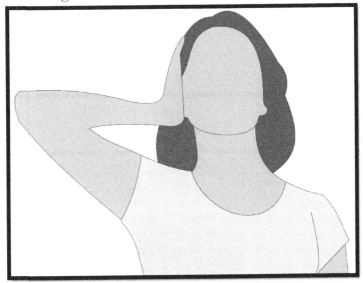

1. Place your hand on the right side of your head on the right ear. Push your hand and head against each other, resisting the movement.
2. Hold for five counts and release.
3. Keep breathing as you perform the exercise.
4. Repeat five times.

Isometric left Lateral Flexion
1. Follow the procedure of Isometric right Lateral Flexion, but this time place your left hand on the left ear.

Fine Tips:
1. Keep the neck aligned with the spine all the time.
2. Stay in your comfort zone while performing these exercises. If the exercises cause pain or discomfort, stop doing these immediately.
3. Remember to breathe normally throughout the exercise.

Seated Neck Stretches

Effect: Stretches the muscles of neck, shoulders and upper back. Relieves neck and shoulder tension and muscle spasms. Improves neck flexibility and mobility. Helps with headaches.

Important: Practice carefully in case of neck injuries.

Start Position: Sitting or standing straight with spine and neck tall, shoulders relaxed, feet on the ground, chin parallel to the floor and hands resting on the thighs.

Steps:
1. Let your head drop to the left side as if to touch your left ear onto your left shoulder. Keep the shoulders relaxed and chest lifted outwards.

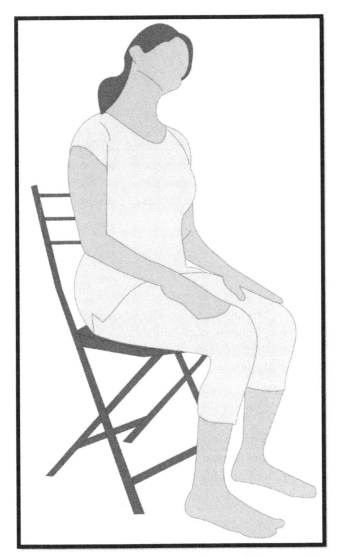

2. Let the weight of your head stretch the muscles on the right side of your neck as the head continues to relax on the left side. Hold this position for 30

seconds to 1 minute, relaxing the targeted muscles and breathing normally.

3. Repeat the above procedure on the other side, letting the head drop on the right side as if you are trying to touch the right ear on the right shoulder. Keep your shoulders relaxed and chest outwards all time.

4. Hold the position in Step 3 for 30 seconds to 1 minute, breathing in a normal manner and relaxing the muscles gradually.

Fine Tips:

1. For deeper stretch in the neck muscles, hang your arms by the side of your body while doing above mentioned procedures. (fig. a)

2. To increase the stretch further, pull with the hand of the side towards which the neck is bent. Avoid over-pulling. (fig. b)

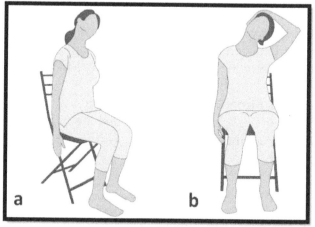

3. This exercise can be done in the standing position also.

CHAPTER 5

Exercises for Shoulder Region

The shoulder joint is the most mobile and hence most unstable joint of the body. This unstable nature makes it prone to injuries leading to degenerative changes which can hamper its movement.

The shoulder girdle attaches to the scapula (the shoulder blade) to the back of the thoracic rib cage (upper back) through large muscles. These muscles help in many vital functions of the body including respiration. They provide support to the upper body helping in the smooth movement of the upper limbs. These upper back muscles are prone to muscle irritation and lack of strengthening due to long sitting hours.

Due to the above stated reasons, shoulder pain associated with upper back and neck pain is a very common condition present in people with a sedentary lifestyle.

The exercises mentioned in this chapter help to strengthen the muscles in the upper back and around the shoulder joints. Practicing these will also help to break the build-up of stress in this area.

Shoulder Rotations

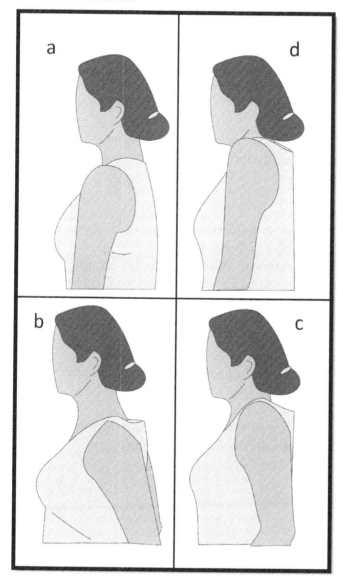

Backward Rotations

Effect: Opens hunched shoulders and chest. Releases shoulder and neck tension. Improves breathing.

Important: Practice with care in case of shoulder and neck injuries.

Start Position: Can be done while sitting or standing with the spine straight, chin parallel to the floor and looking straight ahead.

Steps:
1. Follow the illustration on page 27 in anticlockwise sequence i.e. a-b-c-d-a.
2. Take your shoulders forward, breathe in.
3. Start rotating the shoulders taking them up and behind. Get your shoulder blades (i.e. scapula) together as you move the shoulders behind. Breathe out.
4. Get shoulders back to start position.
5. Repeat this sequence for 10 times and relax.

Fine Tips:
1. The rotation should be slow and rhythmic coordinated with deep breathing.

Forward Rotations

Effect: Stretches your upper back. Releases shoulder and neck tension. Frees up breathing.

Important: Practice with care in case of shoulder and neck injuries.

Start Position: Can be done while sitting or standing with the spine straight, chin parallel to the floor and looking straight ahead.

Steps:
1. Follow the illustration on page 27 in clockwise sequence i.e. a-d-c-b-a.
2. Take your shoulders behind, getting your shoulder blades together. Breathe in.
3. Continue rotating the shoulders taking them up and forward as you breathe out.
4. Get shoulders back to start position.
5. Repeat this sequence for 10 times and relax.

Fine Tips:
1. The rotation should be slow and rhythmic, coordinated with deep breathing.

Forward Arm Stretch

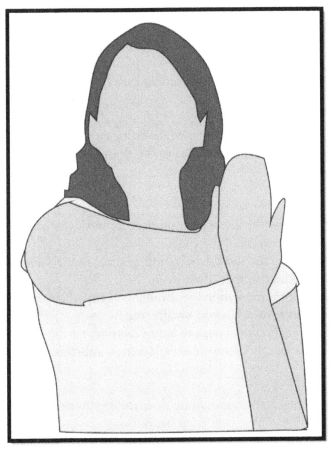

Effect:　　　Opens up shoulder joint and the upper back. Releases shoulder and upper back tension. Stretches arm muscles. Improves breathing.

Important:　　Practice with care in case of shoulder joint and upper back injuries.

Start Position: Can be done while sitting or standing with the back tall, chin parallel to the floor and looking straight.

Steps:
1. Extend your right arm to the side at shoulder level with palm facing forward. Breathe in.
2. Move the arm forward and take it across the chest as if to wrap your chest with your arm. Breathe out.
3. Bring the right hand around your left shoulder blade walking your fingertips towards your upper spine to the extent that it is comfortable.
4. Feel the stretch on the outer side of your right arm, right shoulder and upper back. Breathe deeply into the thoracic spine and upper back, trying to release the stretching muscles and relax.
5. Hold this position for 30 seconds to 1 minute.
6. Repeat the above procedure on the left side.

Advanced Steps:
1. If and when the basic stretch is comfortable, move to a deeper stretch.
2. Give a slight push at the elbow of the wrapped arm, pulling it towards your chest. Feel the increase in stretch on the outer side of the wrapped arm, the shoulder and the upper back.
3. Hold this position for 30 seconds to 1 minute.
4. Breathe deeply into the stretch and relax.
5. Repeat on the other side.

Fine Tips:
1. The stretches should be comfortable and pleasant.
2. Coordinate movement with deep breathing.

Upward Arm Stretch

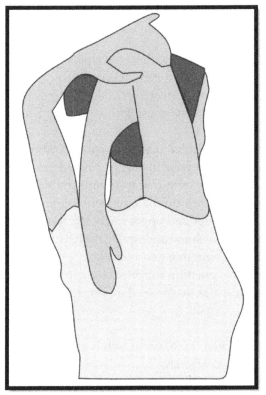

Effect: Opens the shoulder joint. Releases shoulder, upper arm and upper back tension. Lengthens the intercostal muscles.

Important: Practice with care in case of shoulder and upper back injuries.

Start Position: Sitting or standing with spine straight, chest lifted outwards, chin parallel to floor and looking straight.

Steps:
1. Extend your right arm to the side with palm facing up. Breathe in.
2. Raise the arm towards the ceiling and then bend at the elbow till your fingertips reach the spine between your shoulder blades. Breathe out.
3. Walk your fingertips down the spine while breathing in.
4. Feel the stretch on the outer side of your right arm, upper back and the right side of your trunk. Breathe deeply trying to release the stretching muscles of upper back and around the spine. Relax.
5. Hold this position for 30 seconds to 1 minute.
6. Repeat the above procedure for the left side.

Advanced Steps:
1. If and when the basic stretch is comfortable, move to a deeper stretch.
2. Pull the elbow of the bent arm towards the opposite side with your other hand, further walking fingers down the spine.
3. Hold the stretch when it is deep enough and comfortable, preferably for 30 seconds to 1 minute
4. Breathe deeply, trying to further release the stretching muscles of the upper back and around the spine and relax.
5. Repeat for the other side.

Fine Tips:
1. The stretch should be comfortable and pleasant. Avoid over-stretching.
2. Coordinate deep breathing with the stretches.

Backward Arm Stretch

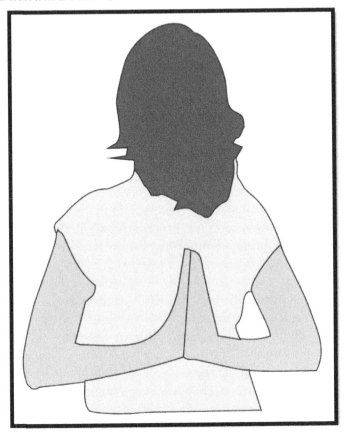

Effect: Opens up the shoulder joints and chest. Releases tension in the shoulders and neck muscles. Reduces hunching of the back making it straight. Stretches the hands and wrists. Frees up breathing.

Important: Care must be taken while performing this stretch in case of shoulder, hand and wrist injuries.

Start Position: Sit or stand with back tall, chin parallel to floor, shoulders relaxed while looking ahead.

Steps:
1. Extend both the arms to the sides making a "T". The palms should be facing forward and thumb upwards.
2. Rotate your arms so that the palms face backwards and the thumb is facing downwards. Inhale deeply.
3. Bend your arms at the elbows and bring both hands behind your back till the tip of middle fingers touch each other with little fingers of both hands pressing against the back. Exhale deeply.
4. Start pushing the middle fingers up slowly. Try to bring all fingers of left hand in contact with fingers of right hand. Slide the fingers up the spine till the stretch is comfortable. Inhale deeply while stretching the muscles of the shoulders, chest, arms and fingers, relaxing them.
5. Hold this position for 30 seconds to 1 minute.

Advanced Steps:
1. For a deeper stretch, press the heels of your hands together firmly once the hands come closer to each other behind your back. You can press the hands further by bringing the fingers together making a *Namaste* (Indian Greeting) behind your back.

Fine Tips:
1. The stretch should be comfortably bearable in all stages.
2. Coordinate breathing with movements, inhaling and exhaling deeply as the chest opens up.

CHAPTER 6

Exercises for Arms, Shoulders & Upper Back

The arms, shoulders and upper back work in tandem with each other. They get strained the most during the long hours of a sitting job. Stretching and strengthening of the upper back, shoulder and arm muscles is a must to have a healthy posture. These exercises prevent the onset of pain due to the excessive straining of muscles and joints in this region.

Exercises mentioned in this chapter help you to strengthen the upper back, shoulder and arm muscles in a matter of few minutes. Thus averting acute and chronic pains and improving your attention span at work.

T Arms Rotation

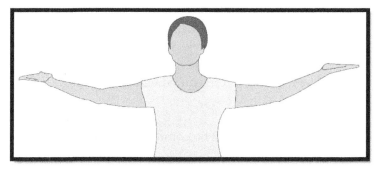

Effect: Opens up shoulders, arms, wrists & hands. Strengthens the shoulders, arms and upper back.

Important: Practice with care in case of shoulder, arm, wrist or hand injuries.

Start Position: Sit or stand with back tall, shoulders relaxed, chin parallel to the floor while looking straight ahead.

Steps:
1. Extend your arms to the side at shoulder level making a "T" with your body. Palms should be facing forward with thumbs pointing up. Keep the elbows relaxed. Inhale.
2. Rotate the arms behind so that the palms face up with the thumb pointing behind. You should feel the movement in the shoulder joint. Hold this position for 10 counts. Keep breathing into the stretched muscles and relax them.
3. Rotate the arms back to the start position so that the palms face forward and the thumbs up. Exhale.
4. Repeat the whole sequence 3 times.

Fine Tips:
1. To further increase strength, you can hold comfortable weights in your hands (stapler / water bottle etc.).
2. Always keep your neck tall, shoulders down and elbows relaxed while performing this exercise.

Triceps Dips

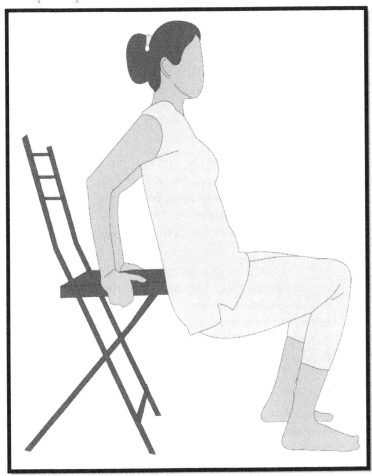

Effect:　　Strengthens the hands, wrists, triceps, shoulder and upper back muscles.

Important:　　Practice with care in case of shoulder, elbow, wrist or hand injuries.

Start Position:　　Sit straight at the edge of the chair with your feet planted one or two feet away.

Steps:
1. Hold the edge of the seat of the chair with your arms by the side of your body.
2. Straighten your arms so that it raises your body up, away from the chair. Inhale.
3. Bend your elbows making your body dip between the arms till your legs are at 90 degrees at your hip joint. Exhale.
4. Re-straighten your arms raising your body back again. Inhale.
5. Repeat 8-10 times.

Fine Tips:
1. Use a stable chair (non-swiveling), preferably rested against a wall.

Biceps Curls

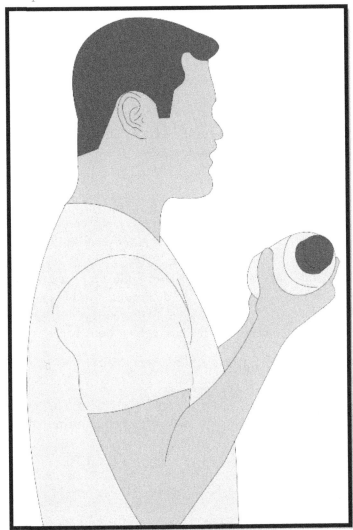

Effect: Strengthens the bicep muscles.

Important: Practice with care in case of arm or wrist injuries.

Start Position: Sit or stand straight with elbows tucked by the side of your body.

Steps:
1. Hold a heavy object like water bottle or handbag in your hands with the object in front.
2. Curl your forearms up. Inhale.
3. Hold the object there for 4-5 seconds. Keep breathing.
4. Roll the forearms down as you exhale.
5. Repeat 10-15 times

Fine Tips:
1. Elbows should always be tucked by side of your body while performing this exercise.

Self-Handshake

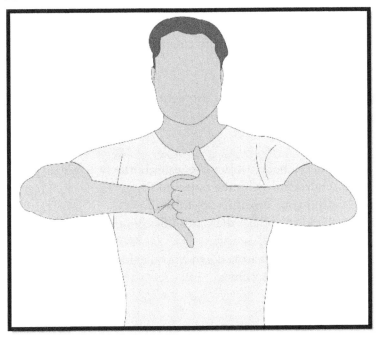

Effect: Strengthens the arms, shoulders, upper back and chest muscles.

Important: Practice with care in case of hand, arm, shoulder, upper back or chest injuries.

Start Position: Sit or stand tall with shoulders relaxed, chin parallel to the floor as you look straight ahead.

Steps:
1. Clasp your hands in front of your chest with the left thumb pointing towards the ceiling and the right thumb pointing towards the floor.
2. Pull hard, resisting the motion of each hand against the other.
3. Keep breathing. Hold this position for 5 counts and release.
4. Repeat 5 times.
5. Switch the hands with the right thumb pointing towards the ceiling and the left thumb pointing towards the floor.
6. Again pull hard resisting the motion of hands against each other.
7. Keep breathing. Hold this position for 5 counts and release.
8. Repeat 5 times.

Fine Tips:
1. Keep the shoulders relaxed; maintain the distance between shoulders and ears all the time, keeping the neck and back tall.
2. The pull should be strong but comfortable.
3. Keep breathing throughout the exercise

W Arms Retraction

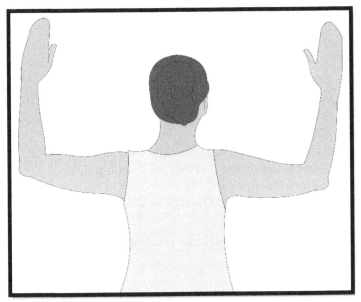

Effect:　　　Opens up the shoulder joints and chest region. Stretches and strengthens the muscles of the shoulders and arms. Strengthens the upper back muscles. Frees up breathing.

Important:　　　Practice with care in case of shoulder, arm or neck injuries.

Start Position:　　Sit or stand with spine straight, shoulders relaxed, chin parallel to the floor while looking straight ahead.

Steps:

1. Extend your arms to the side at shoulder level with palms facing in front. Inhale.
2. Bend your arms at elbows making 90 degrees at the shoulder and elbow joints. Exhale.
3. Take your arms behind bringing the shoulder blades together. Keep breathing deep with the chest outwards, hold for 10 counts and relax.
4. Repeat 3 sets.

Fine Tips:

1. While doing this exercise, keep your neck stretched and shoulders down all the time; maintaining a distance between the shoulders and ears.

CHAPTER 7

Exercises for the Wrists & Hands

The hand is the most distal part of the upper limb, meant for carrying out diverse activities. It is joined to the forearm at the wrist joint. Numerous muscles, tendons, bursae, blood vessels and nerves are artistically placed and protected in this region.

Long hours of working on computers can compromise hand and wrist health. The two most common problems faced today are Carpal Tunnel Syndrome & De Quervain's Disease. Carpal Tunnel Syndrome is the impingement on the median nerve in the area of the wrist that can cause numbness, tingling and eventually pain & cramping in the hand. De Quervain's Disease is the inflammation of the tendons that begin in the thumb and extend to the wrist, causing wrist pain.

The stretching and strengthening exercises mentioned in this chapter helps to maintain the health of the joints and muscles in and around the wrist and hand areas.

Wrist Extensions

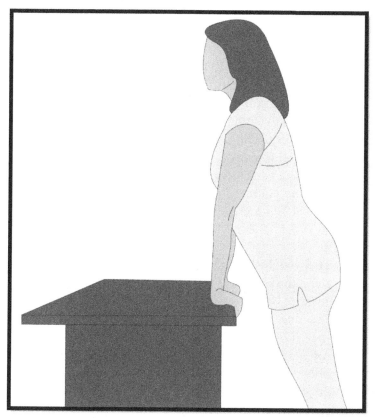

Effect: Stretches wrist flexors, arm & forearm flexors. Strengthens arms and forearms. Prevents Carpal Tunnel Syndrome.

Important: Practice with care in case of hand, wrist, arm & shoulder injuries.

Start Position: Stand tall facing the desk, one foot away from it.

Steps:
1. Grasp the edge of the desk with your hands such that your fingers are facing down and the palm is facing away from you.
2. Keeping the arms straight at the elbows, lean over the hands, feeling the stretch on the front side of arms and forearms.
3. Hold the stretch for 5 counts and release. Keep breathing during the stretches.
4. Repeat 10 times.

Fine Tips:
1. The stretch should be comfortable.
2. Keep the shoulders relaxed while maintaining the distance between the ears and shoulders.
3. You may have to adjust the table height to get the stretch right. If the table is higher than required then you won't feel the stretch in your arms. On the other side, if the table is too short then you may get a strain on your back.

Wrist Rotations

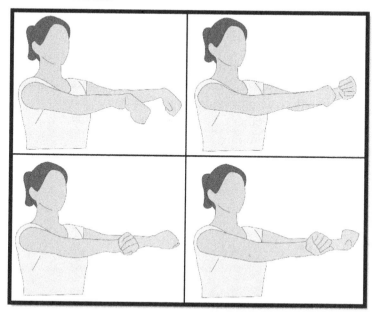

Effect: Stretches the muscles around wrists.
Improves wrists mobility and releases stretched muscles.

Important: Practice with care in case of a wrist injury.

Start Position: Sit or stand tall with arms stretched out in front.

Steps:
1. Make fists and rotate them at wrists 10 times in the clockwise direction.
2. Rotate the fists at the wrist 10 times in the anticlockwise direction.

Fine Tips:
1. Keep your arms & forearms stable while rotating the wrists.
2. Some people find it easier to rotate one fist in clockwise direction and the other fist in anticlockwise direction simultaneously (much like two gears engaged together). You may do exercise this way. Just make sure that you do 10 repetitions for both hands in each direction.

CHAPTER 8

Exercises for Chest

Who doesn't want a well-toned chest? It's a sign of
masculinity in men & femininity in women. A man with a
well-built chest looks strong, confident and may catch the
eye of the opposite sex. No matter what clothes he wears,
it's easy for him to carry his style confidently. For women,
a well sculpted chest with toned and raised breasts adds to
their sex appeal.

The exercises mentioned in this chapter help to tone your
pectoral (chest) muscles. Working chest muscles has the
added benefit of toning and strengthening the muscles in
your arms and upper back (i.e. triceps, biceps and deltoids).

Namaste

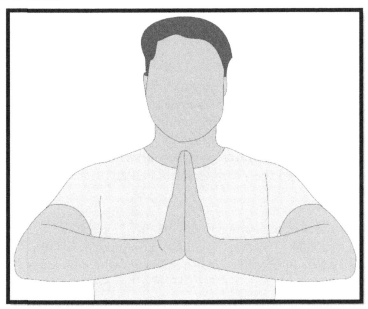

Effect: Strengthens the hands, wrists, arms, shoulders and upper back muscles. Prevents Carpal Tunnel Syndrome.

Important: Practice With care in case of hand, wrist, arm, shoulder, upper back or chest injuries.

Start Position: Sit or stand tall with shoulders relaxed, chin parallel to the floor and looking straight ahead.

Steps:
1. Get your hands in front of your chest with palms pressing against each other.

2. Feel your muscles contract as you press your hands harder. Hold here for 5 counts and relax.
3. Repeat this 10 times.

Fine Tips:
1. Keep the shoulders down throughout, maintaining distance between the shoulders and ears.
2. Keep breathing throughout the exercise.
3. The hands' press should be strong but comfortable.

Wall Push-Ups

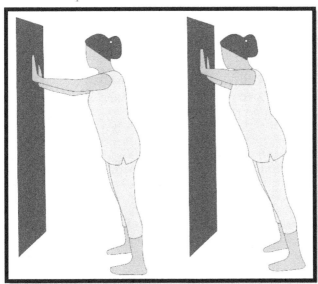

Effect: Strengthens arms, shoulders and upper
back muscles. Opens up the chest. Improves breathing.
Stretches calf muscles.

Important: Practice with care in case of shoulder, arm,
wrist or hand injuries.

Start Position: Stand straight facing the wall, at 1-2 feet
distance from the wall. Feet should be hip-width distance
apart with outer edges of the feet parallel to each Other.

Steps:
1. Stand at a distance of two feet away from the wall.
2. Lean forward until your hands are flushed against the
   wall with both arms parallel to the floor.
3. Bend the elbows bringing your body towards the
   wall. Inhale.
4. Hold here for 5 seconds, keep breathing.
5. Push back to original position. Exhale.
6. Repeat it 20 times.

Fine Tips:
1. Tuck your navel in (engage the core) as you lean
   towards the wall and come back.
2. Avoid shrugging of the shoulders and keep the neck
   tall as you lean into and retract from the wall.

Desk Cat & Camel Stretches

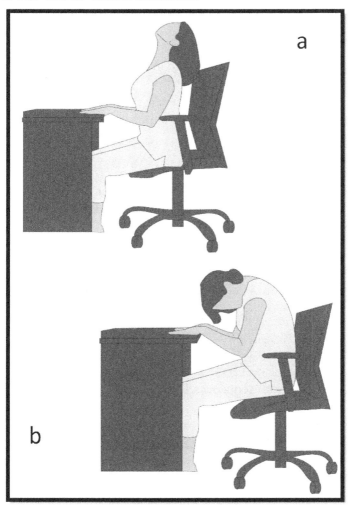

Effect: Improves spine flexibility. Opens up the chest. Frees up breathing. Stretches back muscles, relaxing them.

Important: Practice with care in case of back injuries.

Start Position: Sit with the spine tall, feet firmly on the ground hip-width distance apart, chin parallel to the floor while looking forward.

Steps:
1. Place your hands on the table, shoulder Width apart.
2. Engage your abdominal muscles by tucking navel in by 2 inches.
3. Cat position - Arch your back, stretching away from the desk, opening up your chest in front, extending your neck and taking the chin upwards. Inhale. (Fig. a)
4. Camel position - Pull your abdomen in, making a hump in the back, bending towards the desk, taking the chin towards the chest. Exhale. (Fig. b)
5. Return back to the Start position.
6. Repeat both sequences 10 times each.

Fine Tips:
1. Keep the abdomen engaged throughout the procedure.
2. Deeply exhale and inhale with the movements.

CHAPTER 9

Exercises for Back Relaxation

The back is the support system of the body. It starts from the base of the neck and extends till the buttocks below. It provides support & strength to the trunk along with great amount of movement and flexibility. It comprises of bones, muscles, tendons, ligaments and nerves. Strong back muscles help you to maintain a good posture, reduce back pain and improve functional strength. They also help to keep the spine in a correct alignment. This decreases the abnormal wearing of facet joints, discs and other flexible parts of the spine slowing their deterioration. Strong back muscles also decrease the stress on the ligaments holding the joints of the spine together.

The exercises in this chapter will help you relax back muscles and decrease the build-up of stress which comes from long hours of sitting. This in turn arrests the onset of back pain and muscle stiffening thus helping you to focus more at the workplace. Along with this you develop a Strong and confident personality with a Strong back which Improves your Impression.

Forward Bends in Sitting Position

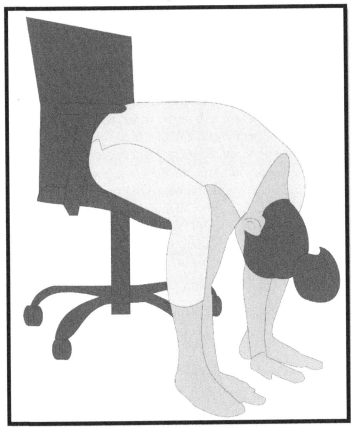

Effect:　　　　Stretches the muscles of the back and pelvic region. Relaxes the neck and spine. Reduces tightness of hip muscles thus improving hip joint mobility. Improves posture.

Important:　　　Practice with care in case of lower back injury.

Start position: Sit straight with feet grounded and placed at a distance little wider than the hip width distance. Knees should be directly over the ankles and toes rotated slightly outwards.

Steps:
1. Place your hands on mid-thigh & stretch your spine. Inhale.
2. Keeping your feet firm, push into the feet; bend your body, vertebrae by vertebrae from the hip region to chest till your hands reach the floor. Exhale.
3. Release your shoulder, neck and head towards the floor. Keep breathing into the hip sockets, spine, shoulders & neck as you relax them. Hold for 30 seconds to 1 minute.
4. Come out of this position by uncurling your lower back first, followed by upper back, then neck & finally straighten your head as you push through the feet into the floor.
5. This exercise can be repeated often throughout the day.

Fine Tips:
1. Sit on a rolled up towel placed on a chair, in case of hip tightness.
2. Always keep the feet firmly on the ground for good balance as you relax your joints and muscles.
3. If your hands don't reach the floor as you bend down, place them over some piled up books or files and relax.

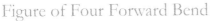

Figure of Four Forward Bend

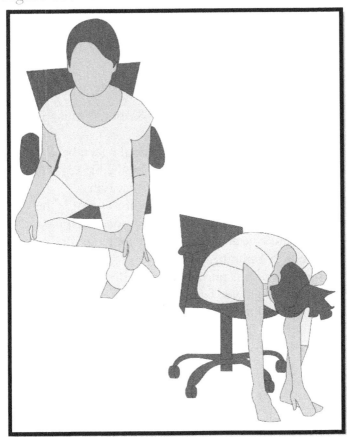

Effect:　　Stretches the muscles of low back and hip rotators. Relieves lower back and hip tension. Improves hip joint mobility. Improves posture.

Important:　　Practice with care in case of lower back injury.

Start Position: Sit with a straight spine, feet firmly placed on the ground, hip-width distance apart. Keep the chin parallel to the floor and look ahead.

Steps:
1. Place your right ankle over the left knee making a figure of 4 with the legs.
2. Stretch your spine straight in this position trying to free your hip joint. Inhale.
3. Let the right knee go down under the effect of gravity opening the right hip joint.
4. Exhale. Bend forward from this stretched position, leading with your chest while still looking ahead.
5. Breathe while stretching and release the spine and hip joints slowly.
6. Exhale and drop your upper body down towards the floor. Feel the increase in stretch in the hip and spine region. Hold this position for 30 seconds to 1 minute.
7. To come out of above position, raise your spine up, keeping it neutral while still keeping the neck and shoulder relaxed. Inhale. Keep pushing through the left foot into the ground to maintain balance.
8. As the spine comes in an upright position, raise the head & look in front.
9. Slowly lift the right ankle off the left knee and place the right foot down on the floor. Exhale.
10. Repeat for the other side.

Fine Tips:
1. The stretch should be comfortable in all stages.

2. Always lead through the spine followed by the neck and head while bending towards or raising away from the floor.
3. Don't push the bent knee forcibly towards the ground with your hand. Let gravity do its job.
4. Relax in the stretched position to get full benefit from it.

L Shaped Body Stretch

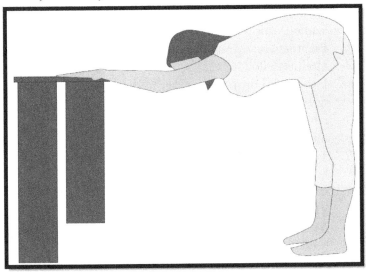

Effect: Stretches the calves, back, shoulder and arm muscles and relieves tension in the same. Opens up the chest. Frees breathing.

Important: Should be done with care in case of shoulder, back & hamstring injuries.

<u>*Start Position:*</u>   Stand straight facing the desk of a height equal to your hip height. The feet should be hip-width distance apart with the outer edges of the feet parallel to each other. The hips & shoulders should be squared (facing forward) and the chin parallel to the floor.

<u>*Steps:*</u>
1. Bend forward and place your hands on the desk, shoulder-width distance apart, making a 90 degree angle at your hips. Exhale. Keep your neck and head aligned with the spine.
2. Give a nice stretch to the spine, pulling the tail-bone away from the crown of the head. Hold this position for 30 seconds to 1 minute.
3. Keep breathing while stretching the calves, hamstrings, back muscles, shoulder muscles & arms and release the stress in them.
4. Come out of the position by pushing into the hands and then straighten up. Inhale.

<u>*Fine Tips:*</u>
1. Keep your weight equally distributed between both feet as you hold the "L" shaped position.
2. Keep your core involved and use your arms to come out of the stretch position. Using only your back muscles would put undue stress on your spine.

Seated Spine Twists

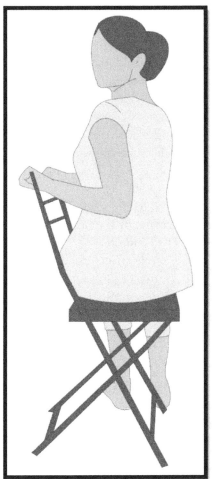

Effect: Stretches the lower back, upper back, shoulder and neck muscles, releasing tension from the same. Stretches the front and sides of the body. Improves breathing & posture.

Important: Practice with care in case of back, shoulder & spine injury.

Start Position: Sit sideways on the chair with thigh parallel to the back of the chair. Sit straight with chin parallel to the floor, shoulders relaxed and spine tall. The legs should make an angle of 90 degrees at the hips, knees and ankles. The feet should be hip-width distance apart. Distribute weight equally between both buttocks.

Steps:
1. From the side sitting position (left thigh next to the chair back), start turning towards the back of the chair.
2. Inhale as you stretch your spine straight from the tail-bone to the crown of the head and exhale as you turn. Keep stretching and turning till you hold the back of the chair.
3. Look behind over your left shoulder in the final position. Keep breathing into the stretch. Hold this position for 30 seconds to 1 minute.
4. Turn your torso back to the start position as you exhale.
5. Repeat the whole sequence on the Opposite side, sitting with right thigh next to the back of the chair.
6. This stretch can be repeated often throughout the day.

Fine Tips:
1. Stretch your spine straight while inhaling and turn while exhaling, giving a nice squeezing action to your torso.

Standing Side Bends

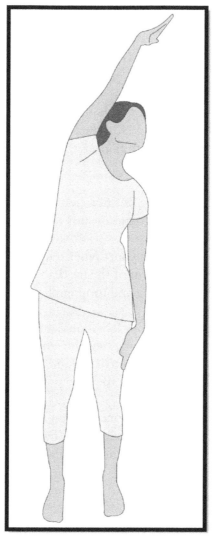

Effect: Stretches the arms and sides of the body. Releases stress in the stretching body parts. Improves posture.

Important: Practice with care in case of arm and back injuries.

Start Position: Stand tall with feet hip-width distance apart and outer edges of the feet parallel to each other. Tuck in your naval and contract your thighs and gluteal muscles (hip muscles). Keep the shoulders relaxed, chest broad and chin parallel to the floor.

Steps:
1. Raise your right arm up with the palm facing the left side.
2. Stretch the right arm up, giving a nice stretch to the right side of the trunk. Keep the weight equally distributed between both feet as you stretch. Inhale.
3. Bend towards the left side with your right fingertips trying to reach towards the ceiling diagonally. Exhale. Feel the increase in stretch on the right side of the trunk.
4. Breathe into the stretch. Hold for 5 counts and relax.
5. Come back to the start position.
6. Repeat for the left side.
7. Repeat 2 times for each side.

Fine Tips:
1. Keep your weight equally distributed between both feet, pushing into the foot of the stretching side as you bend towards the other side.

Standing Backwards Bend

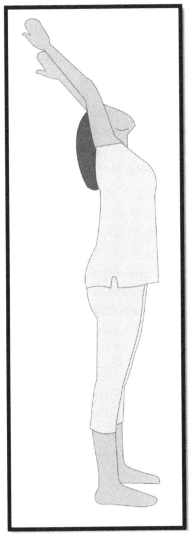

Effect: Stretches the front side of your body. Improves posture. Extends the spine, thus preventing a hunched back. Frees up breathing.

Important: Practice with care in case of back, neck & shoulder injuries.

Start Position: Stand tall with feet hip-Width distance apart and outer edges of the feet parallel to each other. The thighs should be contracted, gluteal muscles (hips) tight and navel tucked in. The shoulders should be relaxed, chest broad and chin parallel to the floor.

Steps:
1. Raise your arms up, with shoulders pulled down maintaining distance between arms ears. Inhale.
2. Bend at your upper back, with the finger tips reaching towards the ceiling. Exhale.
3. Feel the stretch on the front side of your body, shoulders and upper back. Keep breathing into the stretches as you pull yourself up and back.
4. Hold here for 5 counts and relax. Keep deep breathing.
5. Come back to start position as you exhale.
6. Repeat twice.

Fine Tips:
1. Keep weight distribution between both feet equal for the entire duration of stretching.

CHAPTER 10

Exercises for the Abdomen

The abdomen, casually called the belly, stomach or tummy, is the part of the body between the thorax and pelvis. Abdominal muscles play an important role in preventing back pain, improving posture, building functional strength, and maintaining good body balance. There is seemingly no better proof of a physically fit body than properly toned washboard abs.

Abdominal muscles act as an anchor for mid and lower back muscles, thus improving the latter's endurance. Strong abs also decrease the stress on the back after long sitting hours. Weak abdominal muscles make your tummy protrude thus putting more stress on the back. Strong abdominal muscles decrease the exaggerated anterior tilt at the pelvis, which if present can put too much pressure on the lower back discs and facet joints and other flexible parts, thereby accelerating their deterioration. This wear and tear leads to pain, weakness and potential rupture.

Strong abdominal muscles support good posture by helping you prop up your spine, making you look leaner, straighter and more confident. Strong abdomen muscles improve functional strength required during lifting, twisting, bending and getting up from the chair. Exercises mentioned in this chapter would help you tone your abdomen while working in your office cubicle.

Secret Tummy Tucks

Effect: Strengthens core muscles. Help to maintain natural curve of the spine. Improves posterior pelvic tilt and thus prevents increased lumbar curve, which is a common cause of back pain in a sedentary lifestyle.

Important: Should be avoided in case of a flattened lower lumbar curve. Practice with care in case of back injuries.

Start Position: Sit on the chair with back tall and supported, feet grounded and looking straight ahead.

Steps:
1. Take your navel in by 2 inches as you exhale. Your lower back should press against the seat back rest.
2. Hold this position for 5 counts. Keep shallow breathing.
3. Inhale. Release the back press.
4. Repeat it 10 times.

Fine Tips:
1. Take your navel in as you press back against seat back rest, to engage the core.

Chair Crunches

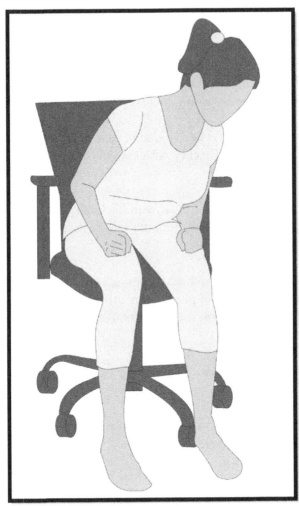

Effect: Tones the abdominal muscles. Improves posture by making the core strong.

Important: Practice with care in case of back injury.

Start Position: Sit tall with your feet grounded and forearms resting on the thighs.

Steps:
1. Take your chest diagonally towards the left thigh. Resist this movement with forearms in the opposite direction. You should feel contraction in your abdominal muscles. Keep breathing naturally. Hold for 5 seconds.
2. Repeat this on the right side.
3. Repeat 10 times on each side.

Fine Tips:
1. Keep your navel tucked in while performing this exercise.
2. Keep breathing shallow as you hold abdominal muscles' contraction.

Chair Swivels

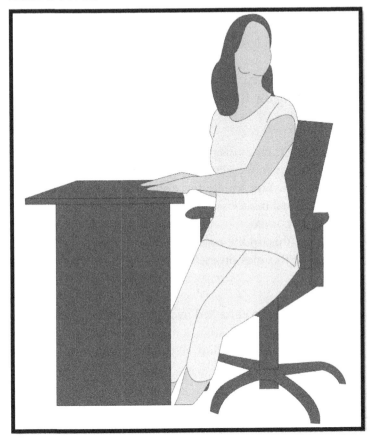

Effect: Stretches muscles of the back, front and sides of your body. Releases tension from the back, front and sides of your body.

Important: Practice with care in case of a back injury.

Start Position: Sit tall on swivel chair with feet floating in the air and tummy tucked in.

Steps:
1. Grab the desk in front of you with both hands.
2. Swivel from side to side. Keep breathing naturally.
3. Repeat 20 times.
4. Can be repeated often throughout the day.

Fine Tips:
1. Keep your spine tall and core engaged (navel tucked in) as you swivel from side to side.

Chair Forward and Backward Movements

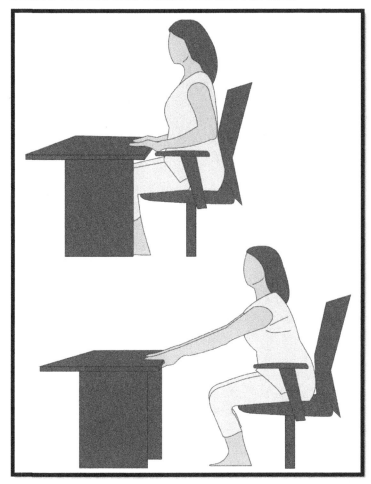

Effect: Breaks the build-up of stress in the upper body, back and arms. Increases core strength.

Important: Practice with care in case of arm, shoulder & back injury.

Start Position: Sit tall on a wheeled office chair with feet floating in the air and tummy tucked in.

Steps:
1. Grab the desk in front of you and roll the chair forward and backward. Breathe normally.
2. Repeat 20 times.
3. Can be repeated often throughout the day.

Fine Tips:
1. Keep your core engaged (navel in) & spine tall throughout the movement

CHAPTER 11

Exercises for Lower Body

Legs are the main part of the human locomotor system. They are the major weight bearing limbs of the body. Having strong legs is a must for daily working, travelling & sports activities. Apart from major functional use, legs have an aesthetic importance too. A firm, well-shaped and toned butt and legs make one look attractive and sexy.

Long sitting hours can weaken your legs and gluteus muscles since you are not using them to hold your body up. With weak gluteal & leg muscles unable to stabilize you, your body is more prone to injuries. Along with leg & butt weakness, long sitting hours lead to tight hip flexors. This can further cause increased anterior pelvic tilt thus impacting your lower back. The result is lower back pain and poor posture while sitting or standing. Long sitting hours can also cause blood to pool in the legs increasing the risk of varicose or spider veins.

The exercises mentioned in this chapter help to tone your hip & leg muscles, improving blood circulation, breaking the build-up of stress and preventing pooling of blood in the lower limbs.

Seat Squeezes

Effect: Releases tension in the hip region.
Improves blood circulation in lower limbs.

Important: Practice with care in case of hip injuries.

Start Position: Sit straight in the chair with body weight
equally distributed amongst both buttocks. Keep both feet
planted firmly on the ground.

Steps:
1. Squeeze your hip muscles as you inhale. Hold for 5 counts.
2. Release the squeeze as you exhale.
3. Repeat 10 times.
4. Can be performed often throughout the day.

Fine Tips:
1. Pressing your back against the seat backrest along with hip squeezes has an added effect on improving posture & maintaining posterior pelvic tilt.

Leg Raises

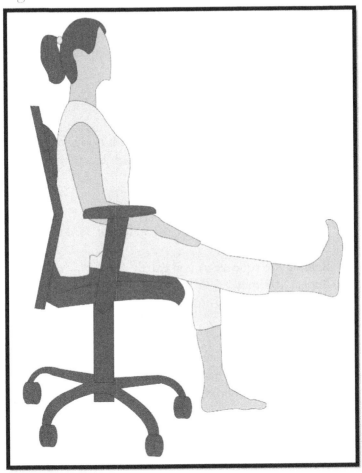

Effect: Strengthens quadriceps (front thigh muscles). Stretches calf muscles. Decreases varicose veins by improving blood circulation in the lower limbs. Improves knee health.

Important: Practice with care in case of knee and ankle injuries.

Start Position: Sit straight on the chair, body weight equally distributed amongst both buttocks. The thighs should be on the seat with the back supported and feet planted on the ground.

Steps:
1. Raise right foot up from the floor to knee level with thighs resting on the seat. You should feel contraction in front of the right thigh and a stretch in the calf. Inhale.
2. Pull the toes of the right foot towards you. Hold it for 5 counts.
3. Slowly lower down the right foot to the ground as you exhale.
4. Repeat on the left leg.
5. Repeat alternatively for both legs 20 times.

Fine Tips:
1. Avoid reclining back at waist level as you raise the leg.
2. Avoid hyper-extending your knee (pushing it backwards) when your leg is in raised position.
3. Leg movement should be slow and rhythmic.

Desk Squats

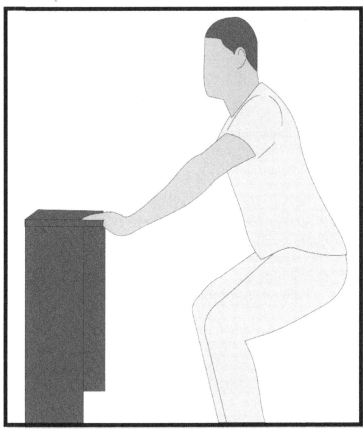

Effect:　　　Strengthens and tones your hips, thighs and lower limbs. Improves posture.

Important:　　Practice with care in case of hip, knee and leg injuries.

Start Position: Stand straight behind the desk, with feet hip-width distance apart and outer edges of the feet parallel to each other. The thighs should be slightly contracted, knees relaxed and buttocks tightened. Tuck the navel in and keep the hips and shoulder squared. The chin should be parallel to the floor.

Steps:
1. Bend your knees keeping the spine neutral and chin parallel to floor. Push your hips down and behind till the thighs are parallel to the floor. Exhale.
2. Hold this position for 10 counts. Keep breathing naturally.
3. Raise your body to the start position, pushing through the heel. Inhale.
4. Repeat 4 to 5 times.

Fine Tips:
1. The knees should never cross the ankle line as you lower your body.

Standing Leg Curls

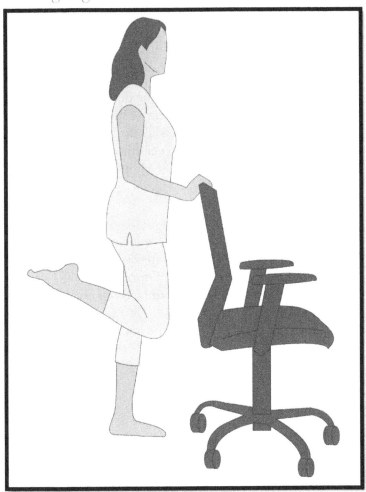

Effect:　　Stretches the front thigh muscles and releases them. Improves posture. Improves blood circulation in lower limbs.

Important:　　Practice with care in case of knee and lower limb injuries.

Start Position:　　Stand tall behind the chair with feet hip width apart. The outer edges of the feet should be parallel to each other. The thighs should be slightly contracted and the knees relaxed. The buttocks should be tightened, with navel tucked in, hips & shoulders squared and chin parallel to the floor.

Steps:
1. Grasp the backrest of chair and bend the right leg up trying to kick the backside of the right thigh with the right heel.
2. Feel the stretch on the front side of the right thigh.
3. Repeat on the left leg.
4. Repeat by alternating legs 20 times. Keep breathing naturally.

Inner Thigh Squeezes

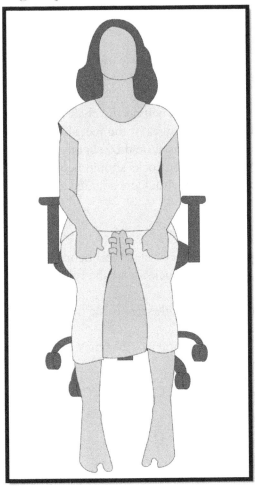

Effect: Strengthens and tones thigh muscles. Relaxes thigh muscles. Improves knee health. Improves posture. Improves circulation in lower limbs.

Important: Practice with care in case of leg Injuries.

Start Position: Sit tall on the chair with body weight equally distributed amongst both buttocks. The thighs should be on the seat with back supported and feet on the ground.

Steps:
  1. Put a bag or sealed pile of papers between your knees.
  2. Press on the bag/papers with your knees and the inner part of thighs as you contract the thighs.
  3. Hold this for 5 counts as you exhale.
  4. Inhale and release the grip.
  5. Repeat 10 times.

Fine Tips:
  1. Squeeze your buttocks and press your knees for enhanced lower limb toning effect.

Tap into Toes

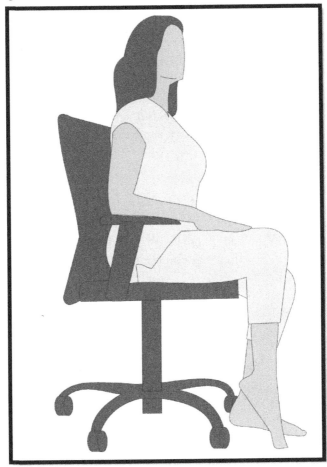

Effect: Relaxes ankle and foot muscles. Improves blood circulation in lower limbs.

Important: Practice with care in case of ankle or foot Injuries.

Start Position: Sit or stand straight with weight equally distributed between both legs.

Steps:
1. Tap your alternate foot toes on the ground, raising alternate heels.
2. Repeat 30 times.
3. Can be done often throughout the day.

Fine Tips:
1. Give a nice stretch to your feet as you tap the toes.

Jog in Your Place

Effect: Improves blood circulation in legs. Strengthens the legs. Relaxes stretched leg muscles.

Important: Practice with care in case of hip, knee, ankle or foot injuries.

Start Position: Stand straight with knees relaxed and buttocks contracted. Tuck the navel in. Keep the hips & shoulders squared and chin parallel to the floor.

Steps:
1. Jog at your place, raising knees high up.
2. Repeat for 1 minute. Keep breathing naturally.

Calf Raises

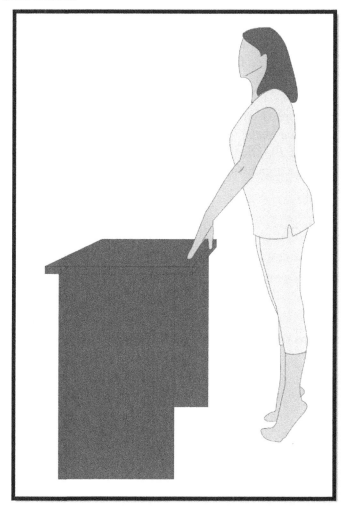

Effect: Tones calf muscles. Improves blood circulation in legs. Reduces varicose veins. Relaxes stretched muscles.

Important: Practice with care in case of ankle or foot injuries.

Start Position: Stand straight behind the desk, with feet hip-width distance apart and the outer edges of the feet parallel to each other. Keep your thighs slightly contracted and knees relaxed. Keep buttocks contracted, navel in and hips & shoulders squared. Keep the chin parallel to the floor.

Steps:
1. Hold the table lightly and raise your body on your toes. Inhale.
2. Feel the contraction in your calves and hold this position for 5 counts.
3. Lower down the heels. Exhale.
4. Repeat this 20 times. Can be done often throughout the day.

Fine Tips:
1. Stand tall and avoid leaning ahead as you raise yourself on the tips of your toes.
2. Avoid hyper-extension of the knee (pushing back of knee) as you stand on your toes.

Standing Leg Raises - Sideward

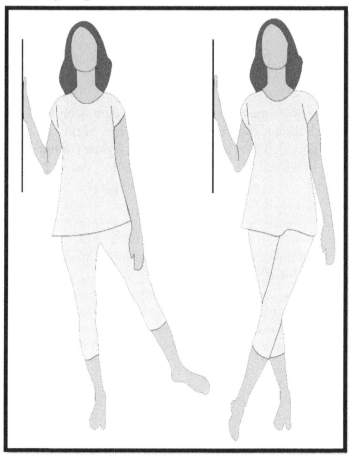

Effect: Strengthens leg abductors and adductors. Improves single leg standing balance. Shakes off tension from the legs. Improves lower limb blood circulation.

Important: Practice with care in case of leg injuries.

Start Position: Stand sideways with your right side next to a wall, about 1 foot distance away from it.

Steps:
1. Place your right hand on the wall.
2. Taking all weight on the right leg, try to balance on the right foot.
3. Move your left leg at the hip joint, sideways, first Outwards (away from right leg), then inwards (towards right leg).
4. Exhale while taking leg outwards and inhale while moving leg inwards.
5. Repeat the above movement 20 times.
6. Change the side with your left side now towards the wall.
7. Repeat above sequence, now moving right leg, 20 times.

Fine Tips:
1. Stand tall as you lift the leg sideward. Avoid bending your trunk on the supporting leg side.

Standing Leg Raises - Forwards & Backwards

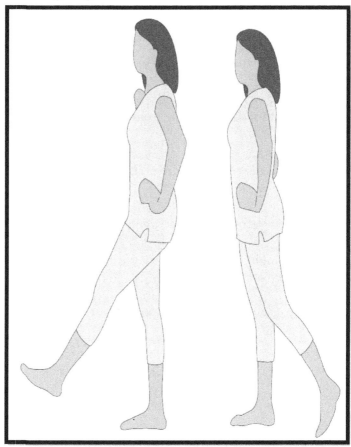

Effect: Strengthens leg extensors & flexors. Improves single leg standing balance. Shakes off tension from the legs. Improves lower limb blood circulation.

Important: Practice with care in case of leg Injuries.

Start Position: Stand sideways with right side next to a wall, about 1 foot away from it.

Steps:
1. Place your right hand on the wall.
2. Taking all weight on the right leg, try to balance on the right foot.
3. Move your left leg forwards and backwards.
4. Repeat the above movement 20 times.
5. Change the side with the left leg next to the wall.
6. Repeat above sequence, now moving right leg, 20 times.

Fine Tips:
1. Stand tall as you move the leg forwards & backwards. Avoid bending your trunk on the supporting leg side.

CHAPTER 12

Shake the Tension Off

Long hours of computer usage fatigues your arms and hands. This affects the efficiency of your work and may lead to stress related injuries and pain in the long term. Hence it's essential to break this build-up of fatigue through repeated rhythmic movements, to relax the strained muscles.

Exercises mentioned in this chapter will help you to release fatigue from strained arms and hands through quick and easy movements.

Fist Punches

Effect: Releases the tension in the arms and shoulder region. Stretches the arm. Opens up the shoulder joint.

Important: Practice with care in case of neck, shoulder, elbow or wrist injuries.

Start Position: Sit or stand tall with chin parallel to floor. Look ahead.

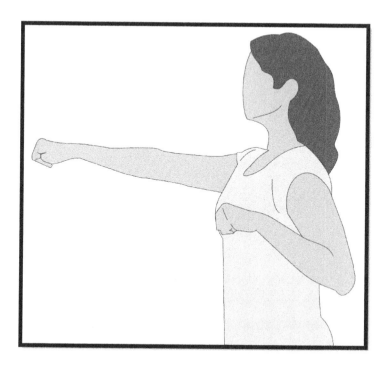

Steps:
1. Raise your arms in front to the shoulder level.
2. Punch your arms in front 60 times alternatively.
3. Breathe in as you bend the arm and breathe out as you stretch it.

Fine Tips:
1. Keep the movements rhythmic.

Flapping Arms

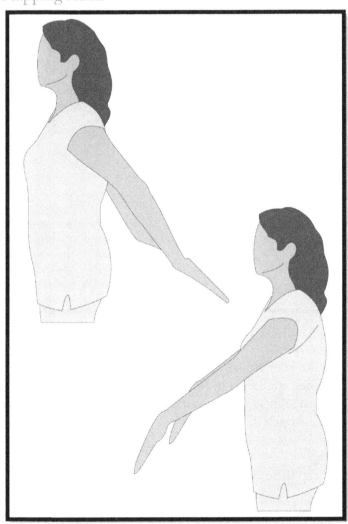

Effect: Releases the tension in the arms and shoulders.

Important: Practice with care in case of shoulder injury.

Start Position: Stand tall with arms by your side, shoulders relaxed and chin parallel to floor.

Steps:
1. Rotate the arms till the palms face behind.
2. Pulse the arms forward & backward 60 times.

Fine Tips:
1. Keep the movements rhythmic.

Axe Movement

Effect: These diagonal movements stretch the arms and upper back diagonally. Thus releasing tension in stretched muscles. Frees the elbow joint.

Important: Practice with care in case of elbow injury.

Start Position: Sit tall with shoulders relaxed and chin parallel to the floor.

Steps:
1. Clasp your hands and bend your arms at the elbows.
2. Rest your clasped hands at your right shoulder. Inhale.

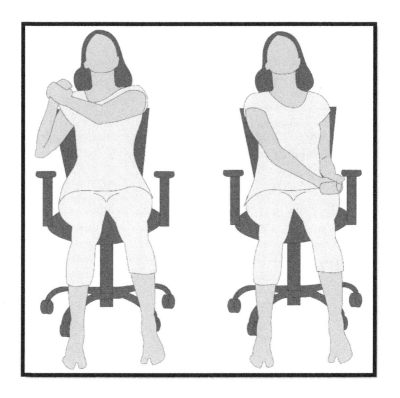

3. Straighten your arms moving the clasped hands diagonally to the left thigh. Exhale.
4. Take the clasped hands to the left shoulder. Inhale.
5. Straighten your arms taking the clasped hands diagonally to the right thigh. Exhale.
6. Repeat the above sequence 10 times.

Fine Tips:
1. Keep the shoulders down and sides of trunk straight as you do the axe movement.

CHAPTER 13

Progressive Muscle Relaxation

Anxiety or stress at the workplace is very common. One of the ways your body responds to stress is with increased muscle tension. The build-up of muscle tension can lead to aches and pains in various body parts, thus affecting concentration levels while working. This is the reigning cause of decreased work output now-a-days.

One quick and easy way to lower this build-up of muscle tension is through Progressive Muscle Relaxation (PMR).

What is PMR?

This is a technique in which you tense a group of muscles as you breathe in and relax them as you breathe out. You work on your muscle groups in a certain order. The muscles are contracted for 4 counts with inhalation and relaxed for 10 counts with exhalation.

Effects of PMR

With PMR the muscles relax and straighten. This helps in opening up tiny blood vessels which were earlier compressed due to higher muscle tension. Improved blood flow to muscles results in the decongestion of the tissues of that area. It provides greater oxygen delivery, better nutrition and more efficient removal of toxins to and from the muscles. It also lowers inflammation and swelling in the acute & chronically injured body parts (especially neck and back) which is normally associated with long sitting hours.

A relaxed body exerts a calming and stabilizing influence on your mind and vice versa, reducing stress and anxiety.

Start Position: Sit relaxed in your chair with back and thighs well supported and feet placed firmly on the ground.

1. _Hands & Forearms:_ Contract your right hand making a fist. Relax and continue relaxing. Repeat the exercise with your left hand. Repeat it with both hands simultaneously.

2. _Biceps & Upper Arms:_ Clench your hands into fists, bend your arms at elbows and contract the muscles on the front of your upper arm (biceps). Relax and continue relaxing. Repeat the exercise.

3. _Triceps:_ Bend both arms at elbows. Contract the muscles of your arms by pushing the back of your upper arms against the backrest of your chair. Relax.

4. Concentrate on relaxing your hands, forearms & upper arms all together.

5. _Forehead:_ Make a frown and wrinkle your forehead. Relax and continue relaxing.

6. *Around the eyes & bridge of the nose*: Close your eyes as tightly as possible. (Remove your contact lenses before beginning this exercise). Relax.

7. *Around the mouth*: Press your lips together tightly and press your tongue to the roof. Relax.

8. *Cheeks*: Smile widely. Relax.

9. *Jaws*: Clench your teeth. Relax.

10. *Neck & Throat*: Push your head backwards while tucking in your chin. Relax.

11. Relax your forehead, jaws, lips, tongue, neck and throat. Relax your hands, forearms and upper arms. Keep relaxing all the muscles.

12. *Shoulders*: Hunch your shoulders to your ears. Relax.

13. *Upper Back*: Retract shoulders. Relax.

14. Relax lips, tongue, neck, throat, shoulder and upper back. Keep relaxing these muscles.

15. *Chest*: Take a deep breath and hold it. Exhale.

16. *Abdomen*: Suck in your abdomen, flattening your lower back against the chair backrest. Relax.

17. *Lower Back*: Contract and arch your lower back away from the chair backrest. Relax.

18. *Hips and Buttocks*: Squeeze your buttocks tightly. Relax.

19. *Thighs*: Clench your thighs tightly. Relax.

20. Relax your shoulders, upper back, abdomen, lower back, thighs and buttocks. Keep relaxing these muscles together.

21. *Shins*: pull your toes towards you. Feel the stretch in your calves and relax. Push your toes away from your body. Feel the calves' contract and relax.

22. *Toes*: Curl your toes. Fan the toes up and apart. Relax.

23. Relax every muscle in your body all together and keep relaxing.

CHAPTER 14

Breath Awareness

Stress and emotional tension at the workplace are not uncommon. As daily stress accumulates in our mind and body, breathing gets strained.

Few changes in breathing pattern due to stress are

- *Over breathing* (Hyper ventilation) that is deep and rapid breathing leading to feeling lightheaded, dizzy, weak or not being able to think straight. You may get chest pain or a fast and pounding heartbeat. You might feel as if you can't catch your breath. This may be associated with dry mouth, muscle spasms in hand & feet, numbness and tingling in the arms or around the mouth.

- *Shallow breathing* (Thoracic breathing) drawing minimal breath into the lungs generally using only the chest muscles (and not diaphragm) reducing oxygen levels in the blood.

- *Paradoxical breathing* is a condition when your chest moves inwards during inhalation instead of moving outwards and you pull your abdomen in as you inhale. This abnormal movement of chest and abdomen affects the breathing pattern and stops you from inhaling enough oxygen. Out of many other causes, stress is a very common cause of paradoxical breathing.

- *Rapid breathing.*

- Breathing through the mouth.

The above mentioned changes in the breathing pattern decrease energy levels, increase physical and mental exhaustion and decrease performance at work.

Know Your Breath / Breath Awareness

Breath awareness is carefully focusing on each stage of breathing as you breathe slowly and gently. It is one of the easiest ways of improving your physical and mental health.

Steps of breath awareness:

1. Observe your breath: Sit relaxed in your chair giving enough space for your abdomen to move in and out. Close your eyes and start observing your breath. Feel the cool air moving in through the nostrils as you inhale and warm air coming out as you exhale. Let the thoughts come and go. Focus only on your breath flowing through your body. Be one with yourself.

2. Practice sectional breathing:
   a. Abdominal (Diaphragmatic) breathing –

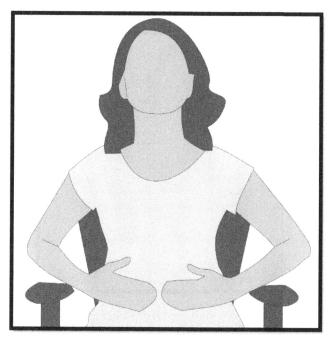

i. Place your hands on your abdominal region.

ii. Inhale deeply & slowly. Your abdomen bulges out with inhalation. Hold your breath for few seconds.

iii. Exhale slowly and completely. Your abdomen is drawn inwards continuously and slowly with exhalation.

iv. Before inhaling again, hold your breath.

v. Repeat this breath cycle 9 times.

There should be no jerks in the whole process. The breathing should be slow, continuous and relaxed.

b. Thoracic (Intercostal) breathing –

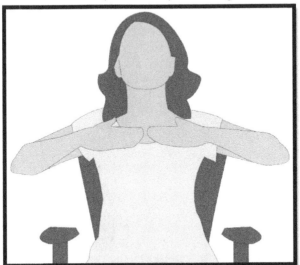

i. Place your hands on the ribs with the tips of the middle finger touching each other.

ii. Inhale deeply and slowly. While inhaling you should feel the chest cage expanding outwards and upwards. The middle finger tips should move apart a little with inhalation.

iii. Exhale slowly and completely. While exhaling relax the chest wall and return to the starting position, with the chest cage moving backwards, inwards & downwards.

iv. Repeat this breathing cycle 9 times. There should be no jerks in the whole process. The breathing should be slow, continuous and relaxed.

c.   Clavicular breathing –

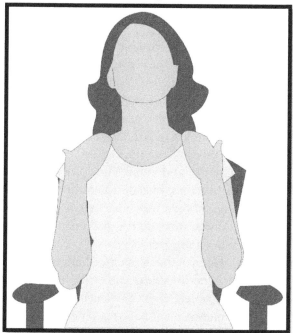

   i.   Place your hands on the clavicular region
         (collar bone).
   ii.   Inhale deeply and slowly. While inhaling
         you should feel your collar bones rising
         upwards and ahead.
   iii. Exhale slowly and completely. While
         exhaling you should feel your collar
         bones and shoulders dropping down to
         the start position.
   iv.   Repeat this breathing cycle 9 times. There
         should be no jerks in the whole process.
         The breathing should be slow,
         continuous and relaxed.

d. Complete / Full breathing - This is the combination of abdomen, thoracic & clavicular breathing.

  i. Sit in a comfortable position; Start inhaling in the sequence of abdomen, chest & clavicle. Your abdomen should bulge, chest cage should expand forward, outward & upwards and the collarbone should get raised ahead & upwards.

  ii. Now exhale in the sequence of clavicle, chest & abdomen. The collarbone should move backward & downwards, the chest cage should move backwards, inwards & downwards and the abdomen should get drawn inwards.

  iii. Once you have practiced enough of guided breathing with your hands on the abdomen, chest & clavicle, you can practice sectional breathing anywhere by focusing on the different sections respectively.

CHAPTER 15

Supported Surya Namaskar

Supported Surya Namaskar is a series of stretching and strengthening movements which involve around 95% of your body muscles. The long hours of a sitting job puts an unusual demand on your posture, muscles and joints. Some areas like the neck, upper back and shoulders become too fatigued due to overuse. The lower limb muscles also become weak due to decreased standing activity.

Supported Surya Namaskar

Supported Surya Namaskar is a quick and effective way of stretching cramped muscles and strengthening unused muscles. Coordinating breathing with the various poses of supported Surya Namaskar has the added effect of energizing your body with positive energies. This makes you more focused, relaxed and energetic at work.

<u>Important:</u>   Should be done with care in case of neck, back, shoulder, upper limb and lower limb injuries.

<u>Start Position:</u>   Stand 1-2 feet away from the desk facing it with feet hip-width distance apart and the outer edges of the feet parallel to each Other. The knees should be relaxed and the thighs and hips contracted. The navel should be tucked in, shoulders and hips squared and the

neck tall. The chin should be parallel to the floor and hands joined in a *Namaste*.

Steps:

1. Raise your arms up, arching the upper back backwards. Keep your shoulders pulled down and the navel tucked in. Give a nice stretch to your trunk as your fingertips reach towards the ceiling upwards & backwards with the arms by the side of your ears. Inhale.

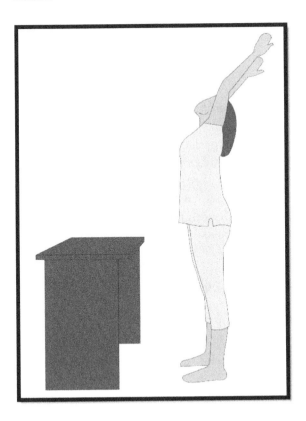

2. Bend ahead at the hip with the feet on the ground. Try to touch your head to the table. You should feel a stretch in the back, behind the thighs and in the calves. Exhale.

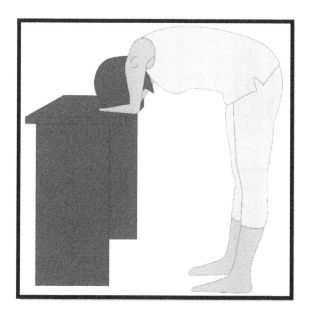

3. Grasp the table with your hands shoulder width apart and arms straight at elbows. Drag your left foot behind in a straight line. Keep the left foot on the ground making 80 degrees outwards. Feel the stretch in your left calf and the muscles behind the left thigh. The right foot stays in front, pointing ahead. The right leg should make a 90 degree angle at both the ankle and knee, with right thigh parallel to the floor. Feel the strength in the right leg. Arch your upper

back and neck upwards trying to open up the chest as you inhale in this position.

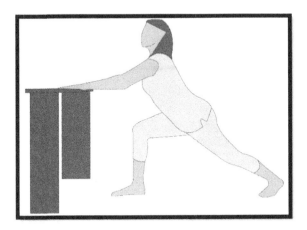

4. From the above position get your body into an "L" position with your hands grasping the desk at shoulder width. Your arms, neck and back should be parallel to the floor with your lower body making a 90 degree angle at the hip. The feet should be planted at hip-width distance with their outer edges parallel to each other. Keep the knees relaxed and thighs contracted. Feel the stretch in your back, behind the thighs and in the calf muscles. Exhale in this position.

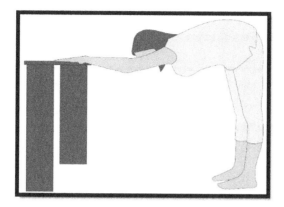

5. Get into a plank from the "L" position with your hands grasping the table shoulder width apart & the neck, back, hips and legs in one line. The feet are planted on the floor hip distance apart. Feel the strength in your arms and a stretch in your calves. Inhale.

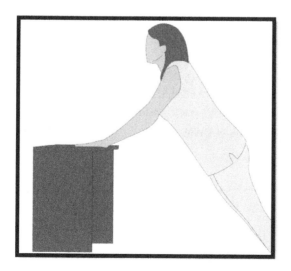

6. Come back into an "L" position (step 4). Exhale.

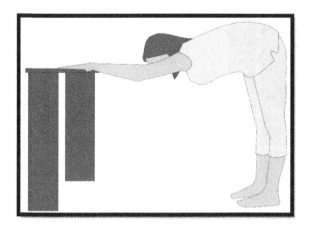

7. From the "L" position, with your hands still grasping the table, drag your left foot in the front in a straight line till the left leg makes a 90 degree angle at both ankle and knee. The left thigh should be parallel to the floor and the left foot pointing forward. Drag the right foot behind in a straight line. Keep the right foot on the ground, making an 80 degree angle. Feel a stretch in the right calf and behind the right thigh. Arch your upper back and neck upwards trying to push the chest outwards as you inhale in this position

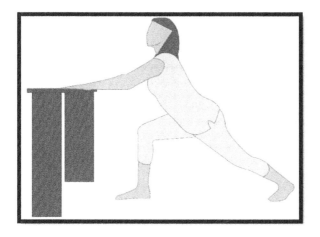

8. Bend over the table as in step 2. Exhale.

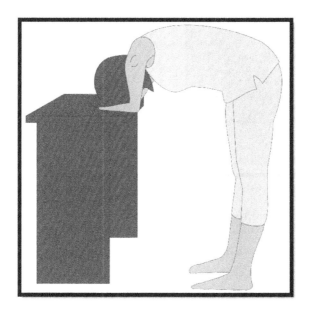

9. Straighten at the hip and stretch upwards and backwards as in step 1. Inhale.

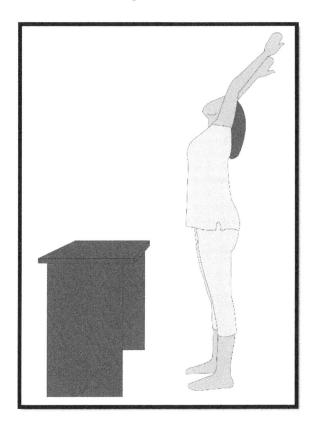

10. Come to the Start position. Exhale

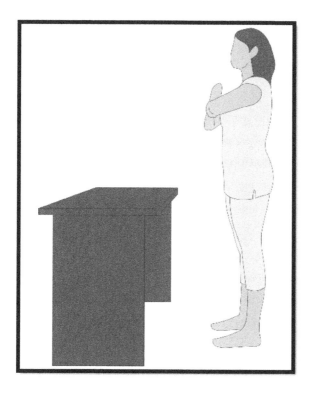

11. Repeat this sequence 12 times.

Fine Tips:
1. Always keep your core engaged in all the postures,
2. The shoulders and hips should be kept squared (facing ahead) in all postures.
3. Transition from one posture to other should be smooth and rhythmic, coordinated with breathing.

CHAPTER 16

Final Tips

Here are my final four tips about maintaining your health while negotiating a sedentary lifestyle in office due to professional compulsions or otherwise

1. Use a Standing Desk: You can buy a desk attachment or place a box on the desk to bring your computer to the standing height. Standing while working gives a break to prolong sitting thus preventing hip flexors shortening, improving posture, increasing calorie burn, improving brain oxygenation and stimulating lymphatic drainage.

   Some people go as far as to use a treadmill as their workstation. But you don't need to do that as long as you are doing the exercises from this book and combining it with intermittent standing work.

2. Take a Quick Stroll: Get up from your work desk and take 3-5 minutes of break every 45 minutes. This can be a quick stretch break, walk to the restroom, drinking water at water fountain or just a stroll around the building. This helps to mobilise the joints, increase oxygenation to brain, and increase attention span after the break. Walk also adds to your daily cardio if done at a fast pace.

3. Walk as you talk: If possible walk as you talk on phone or have discussion with someone that doesn't demand sitting at a place. Take walking status meetings around the lawn. It helps to burn calories and keeps body mobile and active. You can easily burn up to 500 calories a day with 10000 steps.

4. Use an Exercise Ball instead of chair: Sitting on exercise ball while working improves the stability and balance of the body. You have to keep your abdominals engaged while sitting on the ball which improves core strength and hence helps you to have a strong posture. Engaging your core muscles while sitting on exercise ball helps in calorie burn too.

CHAPTER 17

Eye Exercises

Eye specialists advocate the 20-20-20 rule for maintaining good eye health in office. This rule helps to prevent built up of digital eye strain. The rule is very simple – After every 20 minutes you should look away from computer screen for 20 seconds, focusing at something around 20 feet away.

Eye exercises for the office:

1. Palming: Rub your palms vigorously till you feel warmth in your hands. Cup your eyes with the warm hands and feel your eye muscles relax underneath them. Keep the hands on the eyes till they feel warm. Repeat 2-3 times.

2. Blinking: Sit relaxed on the chair with eyes wide open. Blink your eyes 10-15 times quickly. Close your eyes and relax for 20 seconds. Repeat it 4-5 times.

3. Zooming: Sit relaxed on the chair with chin parallel to floor and focus at a point around 20 feet away. Next get your gaze closer, looking at the tip of your nose. Repeat this 10 times.

4. Clockwise and anti-clockwise eye rotation: Sit relaxed with your chin parallel to the floor. Rotate

your eye balls clockwise and anti-clockwise, 10 times in each direction. Then rub your hands till they are warm and cup your eyes with warm hands.

5. Diagonal eye movement: Sit relaxed with chin parallel to the floor. Look diagonally up towards right and then diagonally down towards left. Next look diagonally up towards left and then diagonally down towards right, repeat this 10 times. Then rub your hands till they are warm and cup your eyes with warm hands.

Bonus

I hope you liked the book and have already started doing these exercises in your office. To make it easier for you to follow these exercises at your desk, here is some bonus material.

You can download a printable pdf file that can be pinned up to your softboard for easy reference and as a handy reminder to do your stretches at regular interval. Simply go to:

https://www.fitness-sutra.com/go?id=111145

You can also subscribe to my mailing list to get more tips & motivation to do these exercises.

Your feedback would help me improve this book. Please give me a review on

https://www.fitness-sutra.com/go?id=111256

 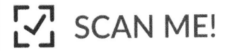

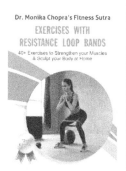

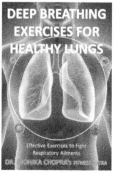

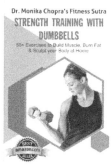

Check out the full collection of books by

Dr. Monika Chopra

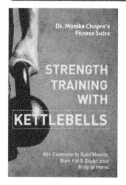

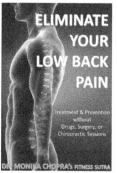

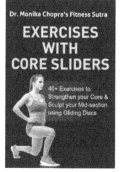

https://www.fitness-sutra.com/go?id=112210

Made in the USA
Coppell, TX
16 June 2023

18171868R00075